Geisla Teles Vieira
Aloísio Jorge Júnior
Millena Q.F. Mazorque

Embryology and Histology Practical Classes Manual

Geisla Teles Vieira
Aloísio Jorge Júnior
Millena Q.F. Mazorque

Embryology and Histology Practical Classes Manual

Textbook

ScienciaScripts

Imprint
Any brand names and product names mentioned in this book are subject to trademark, brand or patent protection and are trademarks or registered trademarks of their respective holders. The use of brand names, product names, common names, trade names, product descriptions etc. even without a particular marking in this work is in no way to be construed to mean that such names may be regarded as unrestricted in respect of trademark and brand protection legislation and could thus be used by anyone.

Cover image: www.ingimage.com

This book is a translation from the original published under ISBN 978-613-9-72506-9.

Publisher:
Sciencia Scripts
is a trademark of
Dodo Books Indian Ocean Ltd. and OmniScriptum S.R.L publishing group

120 High Road, East Finchley, London, N2 9ED, United Kingdom
Str. Armeneasca 28/1, office 1, Chisinau MD-2012, Republic of Moldova, Europe
Printed at: see last page
ISBN: 978-620-7-92346-5

AUTHORS

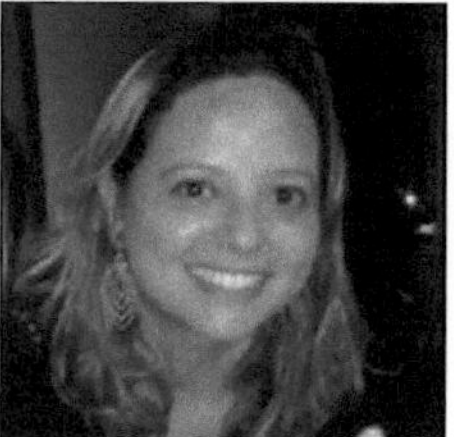

Geisla Teles Vieira

PhD in Applied Biochemistry (UFV), Master's in Pharmaceutical Sciences (UFOP), with a degree in Biological Sciences - BA and BSc (UFOP). She has experience in Biology, Biological Inventory, Pharmacy, Chemistry and Pharmacology of bioactive substances, herbal medicines, Biochemistry of Diabetes and Inflammation. She teaches Morphofunctional Foundations of the Health-Disease Process I and II on the Medicine course at the Piranga Valley Dynamic College (FADIP). She has teaching experience in higher education, teaching the subjects of Environmental Epidemiology, Fundamentals of Biology, Environmental Pollution, Monograph Orientation and Environmental Impact Assessment, and postgraduate experience teaching the subject Biological Inventory.

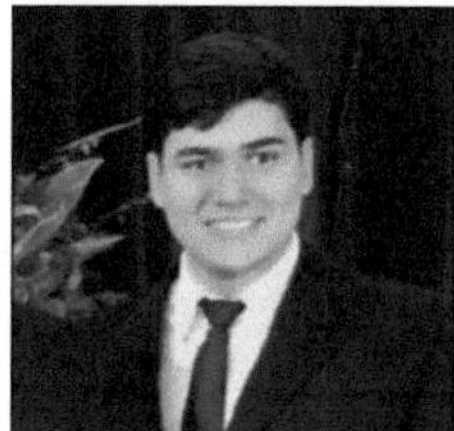

Aloísio de Freitas Jorge Júnior

Graduating in Medicine from the Faculdade Dinâmica do Vale do Piranga (FADIP); scholarship holder of the Institutional Programme for Scientific Initiation Scholarships - PIBIC and volunteer intern for Scientific Initiation at the Medical Sciences Studies Centre - NUMED. Scholarly monitor of the Morphofunctional Foundations of the Health-Disease Process I and II course. Student monitoring coordinator at Faculdade Dinâmica do Vale do Piranga. President of the Academic Surgery League of the Faculdade Dinâmica (LACID). Member of the Piranga Valley Infectious and Parasitic Diseases Academic League (LADIPP).

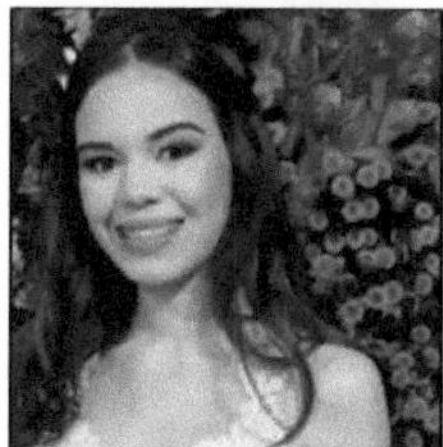

Millena Quinhones Fernandes Mazorque

Undergraduate medical student at the Faculdade Dinâmica do Vale do Piranga (FADIP); voluntary scientific initiation trainee at the Centre for Studies in Medical Sciences - NUMED; former tutor of the subject Morphofunctional Foundations of the Health-Disease Process I (Anatomy and Histology I); director of the Academic Surgery League of the Faculdade Dinâmica (LACID). Research projects: 1) Rationalisation of hospital antibiotic therapy in central nervous system infections. 2) Use of phytotherapics and medicinal plants by the medical population.

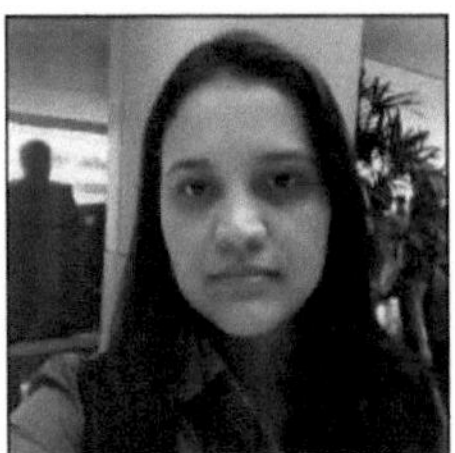

Lorena Souza e Silva

Graduated in Biological Sciences with a Bachelor's degree (2005) and a Licentiate degree (2006) from the Federal University of Ouro Preto. She holds a Master's degree (2009) and a PhD (2013) in Biological Sciences in the area of Structural and Physiological Biochemistry from the same institution. She is currently Research Coordinator, Professor of Undergraduate Medicine, Professor of the Professional Master's Degree in Teaching Health and Environmental Sciences (PROCISA) and Professor of the Lato Sensu Postgraduate Course in Education: Teaching Theories and Methods at the Piranga Valley Dynamic College - FADIP. She has experience in metabolic biochemistry with an emphasis on lipid metabolism, functional foods, hypercholesterolaemia and oxidative stress.

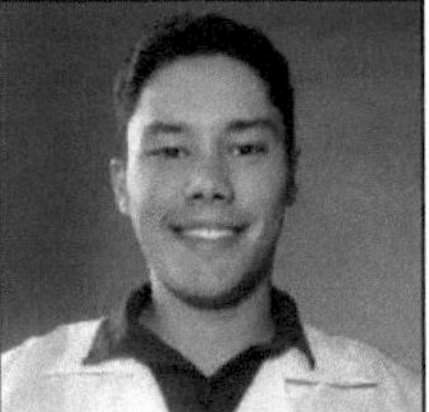

Vitor Carvalho Alvarenga

Graduating in Medicine from the Faculdade Dinâmica do Vale do Piranga (FADIP); voluntary trainee in Scientific Initiation at the Centre for Studies in Medical Sciences - NUMED; director of the FADIP Academic League of Urgency and Emergency (LAUE-FADIP) and the Academic League of Clinical Medicine and Semiology (LACMES); voluntary monitor of the subject Morphofunctional Foundations of the Health-Disease Process IV (Pathology).

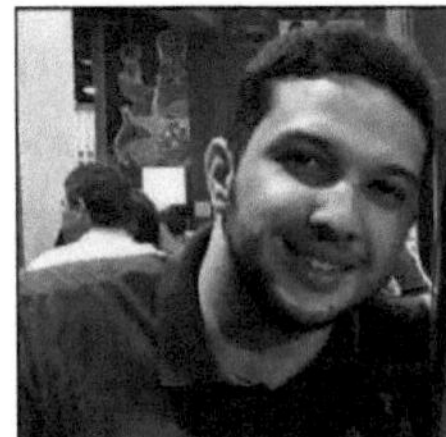

Humberto Jander de Souza

Graduating in Medicine from the Faculdade Dinâmica do Vale do Piranga (FADIP); volunteer trainee in Scientific Initiation at the Nucleus of Studies in Medical Sciences - NUMED; director of the Academic League of Infectious and Parasitic Diseases of the Piranga Valley (LADIPP), the Academic League of Clinical Medicine and Semiology (LACMES) and the Academic League of Anaesthesiology, Pain and Pharmacology (LAADF); member of the FADIP Urgency and Emergency Academic League (LAUE-FADIP) and the

Gynaecology and Obstetrics Academic Medical League (LIMAGO); volunteer monitor of the Pathogen-Human Host Interaction I and Pathogen-Human Host Interaction II subjects (Microbiology and Parasitology).

PRESENTATION

The Didactic Manual of Practical Classes in Embryology and Histology is the result of the work of teachers and students from the Medicine Course at the Faculdade Dinâmica do Vale do Piranga who worked and collaborated in the Morphofunctional Foundations of the Health-Disease Process I subjects.

The aim of the manual is to improve undergraduate teaching by providing students with material to use as a practical lesson guide and study guide. The manual consists of twelve practical lesson plans and their respective theoretical and practical revision quizzes, covering the following subjects: gametogenesis, fertilisation, blastulation, gastrulation, neurulation, animal tissues, bone tissue, lymphoid organs, circulatory and renal systems.

The embryology and histology practicals are aimed at the various courses in the areas of biology and health, with the aim of familiarising students with microscopy techniques and recognising biological structures such as cells, tissues and organs. The study of these structures is important and also applies to morphological analyses in the context of pathology and disease diagnosis.

THE AUTHORS

SUMMARY

CHAPTER 1

PRESENTATION AND PROCEDURES FOR USING THE LABORATORY

INSTRUCTIONS FOR USING THE HISTOLOGY LABORATORY

1. It is compulsory to wear a lab coat and closed shoes and it is essential to follow the practical lessons programme.
2. Class timetables must be strictly adhered to, with students not being allowed to enter 15 minutes after the start of class.
3. Practical class time should only be used to carry out the tasks described in the script provided by the teacher.
4. If any material is damaged, or if something is found to be wrong, the teacher should be informed immediately so that action can be taken.
5. At the end of each lesson, students must turn off and cover the microscope and organise the space they have used it in.
6. Practicals will be considered finished once their results have been approved by the teacher.

EXPERIMENT REGULATIONS

1. Carefully read the script for the lesson you will be taking on the day.
2. Separate the materials you will need for the lesson.
3. Strictly follow the instructions in the script and try to work on your own initiative.
4. To make the most of practical lessons, they should be documented. Drawings should be made in a way that is faithful to what is seen in class, so only sketch what you actually see, without being influenced by materials from the teacher or colleagues. If you don't see any of the structures called for in the script, let the teacher know.
5. Pay attention to the important information given by the teacher and make the appropriate notes. Drawings should contain the names of the structures, and/or legends, as well as appropriate explanations so that they can be used as an aid in future reference.
6. At the end of each chapter there will be exercises for you to answer, which you can discuss with your colleagues on the bench or refer to the texts in the lectures. The questions should be answered on your own at first and corrected when the teacher presents the answers.
7. After using the lab materials, put them in the place indicated by the teacher.

GOOD LABORATORY PRACTICE

1. Eating, drinking and smoking are not allowed in the laboratory;
2. When you enter the laboratory, look for sinks, rubbish bins and suitable disposal areas;
3. Hands should be washed thoroughly before and after procedures;
4. Long hair should be tied back or capped to avoid contact with samples and substances;
5. Contact lenses can make it easier for infectious agents to remain on the mucosa, so their use is contraindicated in the laboratory environment;
6. The use of mascara on the eyes spoils the microscope lens, so students should remove their make-up before classes;
7. Keep your nails well cut;
8. Personal belongings should not be kept inside laboratories;
9. Jokes, side conversations and other distractions should be avoided to prevent laboratory accidents;
10. Before starting any procedure, organise the laboratory and the materials that will be used;
11. Materials on the bench and laboratory apparatus must be properly labelled;
12. Do not smell or taste samples of infectious agents and chemicals from the laboratory
13. Avoid sudden movements when handling samples;
14. If you have any doubts about the procedure or the material used, consult the teacher;
15. Don't scratch worktops and always dispose of rubbish in the appropriate bins.

When you leave the laboratory, leave it clean and organised;

16. In the event of accidents, notify the teacher immediately.

CHAPTER 2

GAMETOGENESIS

SLIDE: OVARY - HE

The ovaries are organs belonging to the female reproductive system. They look like almonds and are approximately 1 cm thick, 1.5 cm wide and 3 cm long. They are lined by a germinal epithelium and just below this is the tunica albuginea.

Below the tunica is the cortex, characterised by occupying the periphery of the organ, being made up of dense connective tissue and containing the ovarian follicles. The composition of this region is detailed below:

- Stroma: Connective tissue and ovarian follicles in various stages of development:
- Primordial Follicles: Found in large numbers. Made up of: A primary oocyte and a layer of flattened follicle cells.
- Primary Follicles: Start of follicular fluid secretion. Formation of fluid-filled cavities. Cells take on a cubic to prismatic shape. Formation of the zona pellucida: Separates the oocyte from the follicular cells. Internal tissue: Vascularised inner cell layer. External tissue: External cell layer resembling stromal cells. Fibrous connective tissue.
- Secondary Follicle: Formation of the antrum (single cavity). Formation of the cumulus oophorus. Ovocyte attached to one end of the antrum. Ovocyte attached to a cluster of cells Formation of the Corona Radiata. Layer of follicular cells. Immediately surrounds the oocyte. Remains attached after ovulation.
- Mature (or Graafian) follicle: Much larger in size. Ready for ovulation

In addition to the cortex, the ovary has a medulla which is located in its innermost region and is made up of a rich vascular network amidst loose connective tissue.

ACTIVITIES

1. Under a 4X objective, make a schematic drawing of the ovary, identifying the cortical region and the medullary region.

2. Under a 10X objective, identify the following regions in the mature follicle: oocyte II, zona pellucida, follicular antrum, thecae, Cumullus oophorus and Corona radiata.

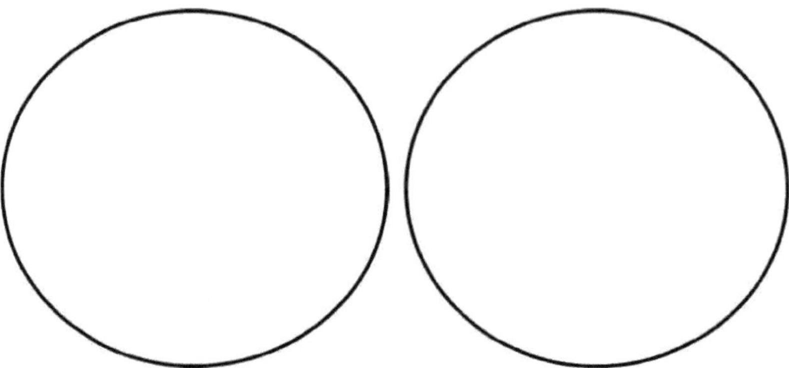

SLIDE: TESTIS - EPIDIDYMIS - HE

Each testicle is an oval organ contained in its own separate compartment inside the scrotum. Its dense connective tissue capsule, the tunica albuginea, is thickened in the testicular mediastinum, from which septa emerge. This tunic is defined as a layer situated just below the serosa, made up of dense connective tissue that divides the testicle into lobes.

The lobules contain approximately 1-4 seminiferous tubules which are structures lined with stratified germinal epithelium containing spermatogenic lineage cells and Sertoli cells - whose functions are to support and nourish the sperm, secrete proteins, provide a haematotesticular barrier, phagocytose and produce anti-mullerian hormone. In addition to these cells, the peritubular connective tissue also contains Leydig cells whose function is to produce testosterone.

The epididymis, in turn, contains the epididymal duct, which is responsible for transporting intratesticular sperm to the penis. This duct has structures known as stereocilia on its surface. The epithelium lining these ducts has an absorptive and digestive action on sperm waste. In addition, the presence of smooth muscle cells helps transport the fluid containing the sperm due to their contractility.

ACTIVITIES

1. Using a 4X objective, identify and draw a schematic of the seminiferous tubules and the spermatozoa in the lumen.
2. Under a 10X objective, identify and make a schematic drawing of the epididymis and its stereocilia located in the epithelium.

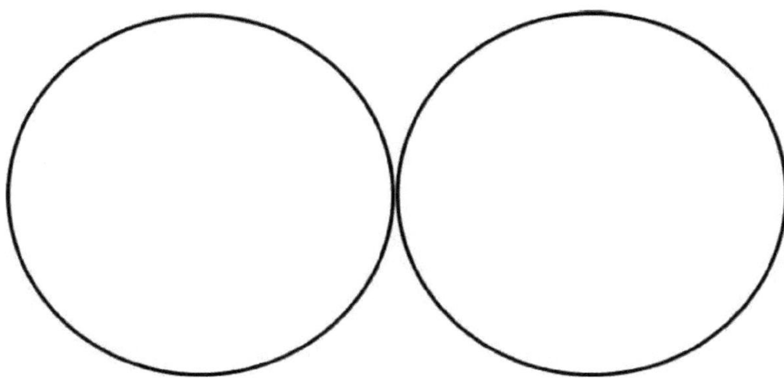

QUESTIONNAIRE

1) Why do we study human embryology? Does it have any practical value in medicine and other health sciences?

2) What are the stages of human development?

3) What is the importance of gametogenesis in human development?

4) What is the function of follicle cells?

5) What is the role of the corona radiata and zona pellucida in the fertilisation process?

CHAPTER 3

EMBRYOLOGY: FERTILISATION - BLASTULA

First Week of Embryonic Development

For fertilisation to occur, the oocyte and the spermatozoon must come together. This union forms the zygote, a highly specialised cell that will give rise to the embryo. During this process many important events must take place, such as the passage of the sperm through the corona radiata present in the oocyte, the penetration of the sperm into the zona pellucida, the joining of the plasma membranes of the sperm and oocyte, the completion of the second meiotic division, the formation of the female and male pro-nuclei and, finally, the mitotic division.

After all the processes that make up fertilisation have taken place, the zygote undergoes successive mitotic divisions characterising cleavage and remains surrounded by the zona pellucida. At this stage, the cells are called blastomeres. When there are approximately 12 to 35 blastomeres, the conceptus is called a morula.

Internally, the morula has cells called the embryoblast and these are surrounded by the trophoblast (flattened blastomeres). The embryoblast will give rise to the embryo, while the trophoblast will give rise to the placenta. When the morula enters the uterus, the blastocyst cavity is formed due to the passage of uterine fluid into the cell mass. During this stage, the embryo is called a blastocyst.

In order for the blastocyst to be born in the endometrium, the zona pellucida that covered it undergoes degeneration. At the moment of nidation, the trophoblast proliferates and transforms into the cytotrophoblast and syncytiotrophoblast. The cytotrophoblast is formed by the inner layer of cells, whose function is to produce new trophoblastic cells towards the syncytiotrophoblast. The outermost layer, the syncytiotrophoblast, has the function of carrying out cell expansion, i.e. expanding the placenta.

At the end of the first week, the hypoblast is formed, which consists of a layer of cuboidal cells, facing towards the blastocyst cavity.

Second Week of Embryonic Development

During this stage, the nidation of the blastocyst takes place and the bilaminar embryonic disc appears. This disc, made up of two layers called the epiblast and the hypoblast, is responsible for giving rise to the tissues and organs of the conceptus. The epiblast is a thicker layer made up of cylindrical cells facing the amniotic cavity, while the hypoblast is a thinner layer made up of cubic cells facing the coelomic cavity.

At the same time, the amniotic cavity appears in the embryoblast. The cells in this cavity (amnioblasts) will give rise to the amnion. The epiblast is responsible for forming the floor of the amniotic cavity, while the hypoblast forms the roof of the exocelomic cavity. The exocelomic membrane and the exocelomic cavity will form the primary umbilical vesicle. The outermost cells of this vesicle form the extraembryonic mesoderm.

After the formation of these structures, cavities appear in the syncytiotrophoblast called lacunae. The lacunae are occupied by a material originating from the mixture of maternal blood with cellular components from the uterine glands, which are responsible for nourishing the embryo. While this is happening, extraembryonic coelomic spaces appear inside the extraembryonic medoserma. These spaces join together to form the extraembryonic coelom and, consequently, cause the primary umbilical vesicle to shrink in size and give rise to the secondary umbilical vesicle.

In the second week, especially towards the end, the chorionic sac develops. At this stage, the extraembryonic coelom promotes divisions in the extraembryonic mesoderm, giving rise to two layers: extraembryonic somatic mesoderm and extraembryonic splanchnic mesoderm. These mesoderms have the function of lining the trophoblast/amnion and lining the umbilical vesicle, respectively. Finally, the chorion, responsible for originating the wall of the chorionic sac, is formed by the extraembryonic somatic mesoderm and the two layers of trophoblast.

ACTIVITIES

1. Draw a diagram of the segmentation sequence of the zygote up to the stage of 8 blastomeres. Identify each part of the drawing.

2. Make a schematic drawing of an embryonic model, identifying: zona pellucida, 1st and 2nd polar corpuscles, male and female pro-nuclei.

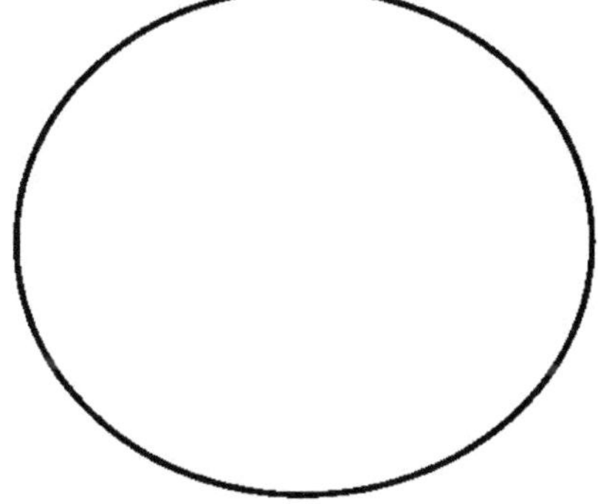

3. In the drawing below, identify the blastocele, trophoblast and embryoblast regions.

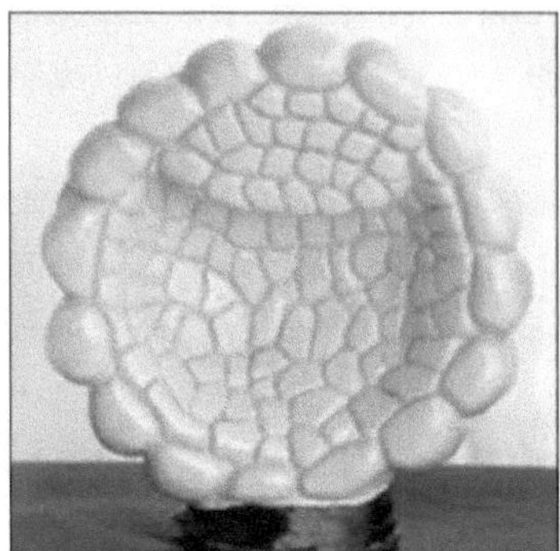

4. Make a schematic drawing of the morula.

5. Which plaster model represents the moment of fertilisation? Make a schematic drawing.

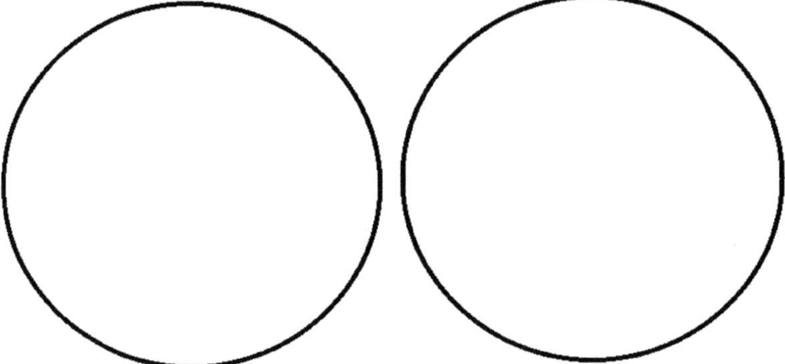

QUESTIONNAIRE

1) What are the main events that take place during fertilisation?
2) Name one function of the corona radiata and one function of the zona pellucida.
3) Explain the cleavage stage.
4) Differentiate between embryoblast and trophoblast, emphasising their functions.
5) Differentiate between cytotrophoblast and syncytiotrophoblast, emphasising their functions.
6) Differentiate between hypoblast and epiblast, emphasising their functions.
7) What is the location and function of the gaps?
8) Name the main events of the blastula.
9) Relate the function of hyaluronidase to embryonic development:

CHAPTER 4

EMBRYOLOGY: GASTRULATION AND NEURULATION

Third Development Week

During the third week, the process responsible for transforming the bilaminar embryonic disc into a trilaminar disc takes place, called gastrulation. The three germ layers give rise to the ectoderm, endoderm and mesoderm. This process begins with the appearance of the primitive streak, a linear band that forms due to the multiplication and migration of cells from the epiblast to the median region of the embryonic disc.At the cranial end of the primitive streak, the primitive node is formed, later the primitive groove, and finally a depression in the node called the primitive fossa. After the formation of these structures, cells from the epiblast migrate through the primitive streak and primitive furrow, giving rise to the endoderm and mesoderm. Until about the fourth week, the mesoderm is produced intensively by the primitive streak. After this period, the primitive streak suffers a significant decrease and the mesoderm begins to produce less.

The next structure to be formed is called the notochordal process. This process is originated by mesenchymal cells from the node and the primitive fossa that have migrated to form the cellular cord. This structure grows cephalad, through the notochordal canal, between the ectoderm and the endoderm until it reaches the precordal plate. During this process, the oropharyngeal membrane (marks the posterior area of the oral cavity), cardiogenic area (primordium of the heart) and cloacal membrane (marks the posterior area of the anus) appear.Therefore, the notochord is an important structure originating in gastrulation, as it provides a basis for the growth of the axial skeleton, delimits the axis of the embryo and designates the area of the future vertebral bodies. Around this structure, the vertebral column develops and, consequently, the notochord undergoes degenerations, but remains in the form of the nucleus pulposus present in the intervertebral discs.

Fourth Development Week

During neurulation, the neural plate, neural folds and neural tube are formed. The neural plate is formed from the embryonic ectoderm, which gives rise to the central nervous system and other structures. Approximately 18 days later, the neural plate invaginates around its central axis and gives rise to the neural groove, which contains neural folds. These folds are the beginnings of the encephalon and, in order to form the neural tube, they begin a process of approximation and fusion. After fusion, the neural tube is completely separated from the ectoderm. Throughout the formation of the neural tube, neuroectodermal cells detach from the neural folds to form the neural crest. The neural crest is located between the ectoderm and the neural tube, dorsolaterally to the neural tube. Its cells differentiate into other cell types and structures such as spinal ganglia and ganglia of the autonomic nervous system, peripheral nerve sheaths, pia mater and arachnoid.The intraembryonic mesoderm gives rise to the paraxial mesoderm which is continuous with the intermediate mesoderm, and from this the lateral mesoderm is formed. The paraxial mesoderm forms structures called somites that are located on each side of the neural tube, whose function is to form the axial skeleton and its muscles, as well as the neighbouring dermis.Another important structure formed during neurulation is the intraembryonic coelom. This coelom initially originates as coelomic spaces located in the lateral mesoderm and the cardiogenic mesoderm, which later fuse. Thus, the intraembryonic coelom divides the lateral mesoderm into the somatopleura and splanchnopleura. The somatopleura is the somatic or parietal layer that establishes contact with the extraembryonic mesoderm lining the amnion, while the splanchnopleura is the splanchnic or visceral layer that establishes contact with the extraembryonic mesoderm lining the umbilical vesicle. It is during the third week that the processes of vasculogenesis and angiogenesis begin. The cells responsible for blood vessel formation are called angioblasts and consist of a specialised type of epithelial cell.

ACTIVITIES

1. Look at the plaster model below. Make captions indicating: endometrium, maternal vacuoles, syncytiotrophoblast, hypoblast, epiblast.

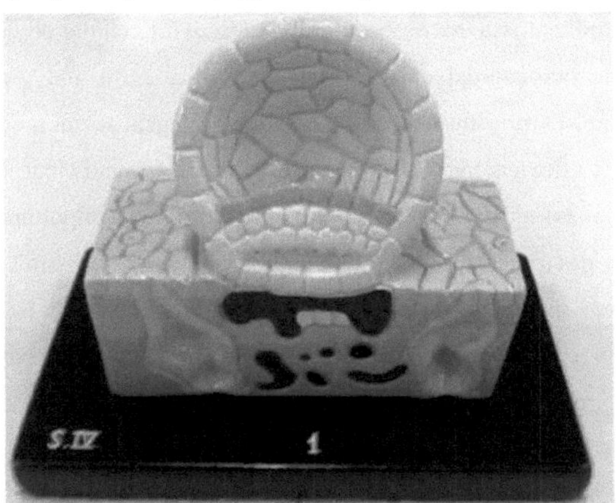

2. Identify the embryonic components on the models and make the legends.

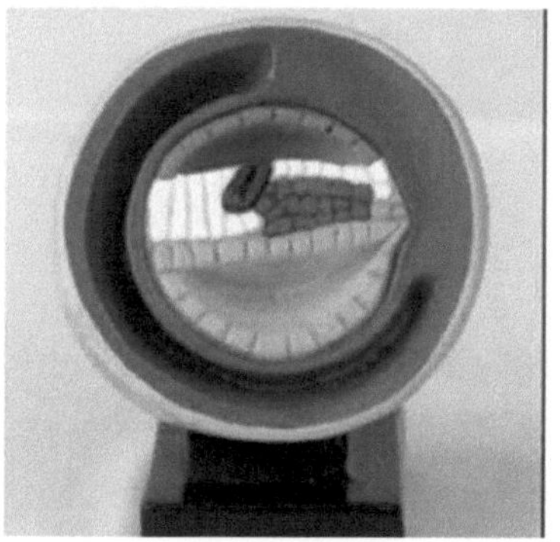

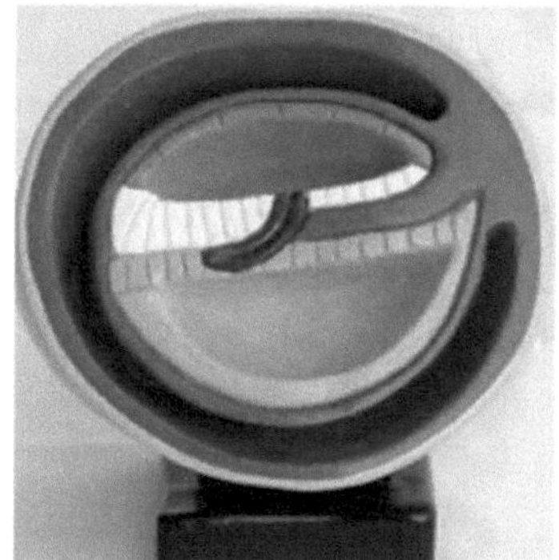

3. Identify the embryonic components on the model and make the legends.

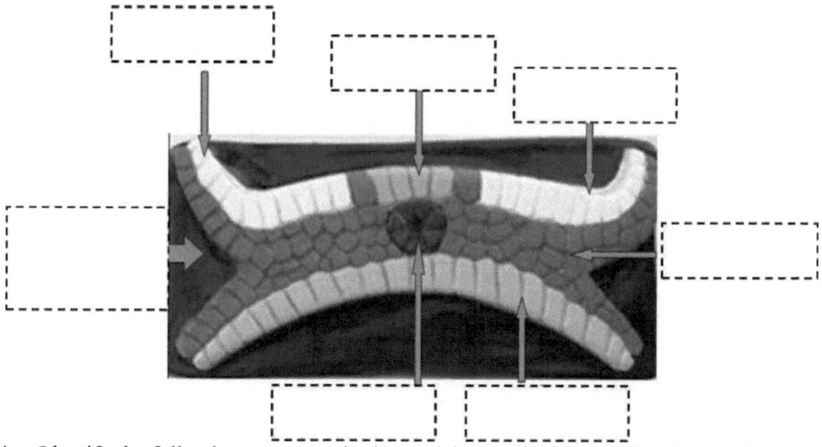

4. Identify the following structures in the model: neural folds, somites, intraembryonic coelom and notochord.

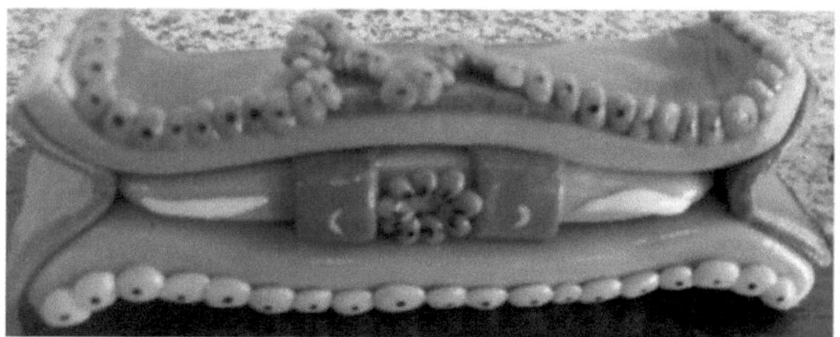

QUESTIONNAIRE

1) Name the three main events of gastrulation.
2) What are the functions of the notochord?
3) What are the main structures formed during neurulation?
4) Explain the formation of the neural plate and neural crest and mention their functions.

6) What are somites and what is their function?

7) Name the function of the somatopleura and splanchnopleura.

CHAPTER 5

ANIMAL TISSUES: EPITHELIAL AND CONNECTIVE

Epithelial tissue

Epithelial tissue is made up of cells that line surfaces or cavities and cells responsible for secretion, with little extracellular matrix. This tissue has several functions, the main ones being: lining and secretion. Lining is associated with protection, absorption and perception. Secretion can be carried out by epithelial lining cells or by more complex structures such as glands.

Epithelial cells are supported by a layer of connective tissue, also called the basal lamina. These cells have portions or poles that vary according to their surface. On the surface facing the connective tissue, the apical surface, the portion is called the basal portion/pole. On the surface facing the cavity, there is the apical portion/pole. Surfaces that are in contact with other epithelial cells are called lateral or even basolateral surfaces. These surfaces can have specialisations such as interdigitations, occlusion junctions, adhesion junctions, communicating junctions, microvilli, stereocilia, cilia and flagella.

This tissue contains juxtaposed polyhedral cells that are joined to each other by specialised structures called intercellular junctions. It can be divided into lining epithelial tissue and glandular epithelial tissue. Lining epithelial cells can have many shapes: columnar or prismatic, pavement-like (keratinised or non-keratinised), cubic, and transitional. In addition, the lining epithelium can be classified according to the number of cell layers it has: simple (one layer), pseudostratified (cells in the same layer, but with nuclei at different heights) and stratified (two or more layers).

The glandular epithelium has cells that have a secretory function. These cells can synthesise, store and eliminate various substances such as proteins, carbohydrates and lipids. Glands can be categorised as exocrine and encocrine. Exocrine glands secrete their material into surfaces or cavities, while endocrine glands secrete their material into the bloodstream.

Connective tissue

Connective tissue has the function of providing support to the body through the extracellular matrix. The matrix is made up of collagen fibres and other macromolecules, which form the fundamental substance. As well as providing support to the tissue, this substance also has other important functions such as reserving growth factors responsible for cell proliferation.

The cells that make up connective tissue are quite varied, including fibroblasts, chondrocytes, osteocytes, plasma cells, lymphocytes, eosinophils, neutrophils, macrophages, mast cells, basophils and fat cells. Fibroblasts, the most common cells found in connective tissue, are mainly responsible for synthesising collagen and elastin. They also synthesise growth factors. When they are in intense activity, they have a large, basophilic cytoplasm, an ovoid nucleus and a large number of organelles such as rough endoplasmic reticulum and the Golgi complex.

ACTIVITIES

LAMINA: Thin skin

1. Under a 10X objective, identify the epithelial tissue and connective tissue on the slide and make a schematic drawing.
2. Under a 40X objective, make a schematic drawing of the epithelial tissue, highlighting the juxtaposition of the cells, the stratification of the tissue and the keratin.
3. Under a 40X objective, identify and make a schematic drawing of blood vessels and fibroblast nuclei in the connective tissue:

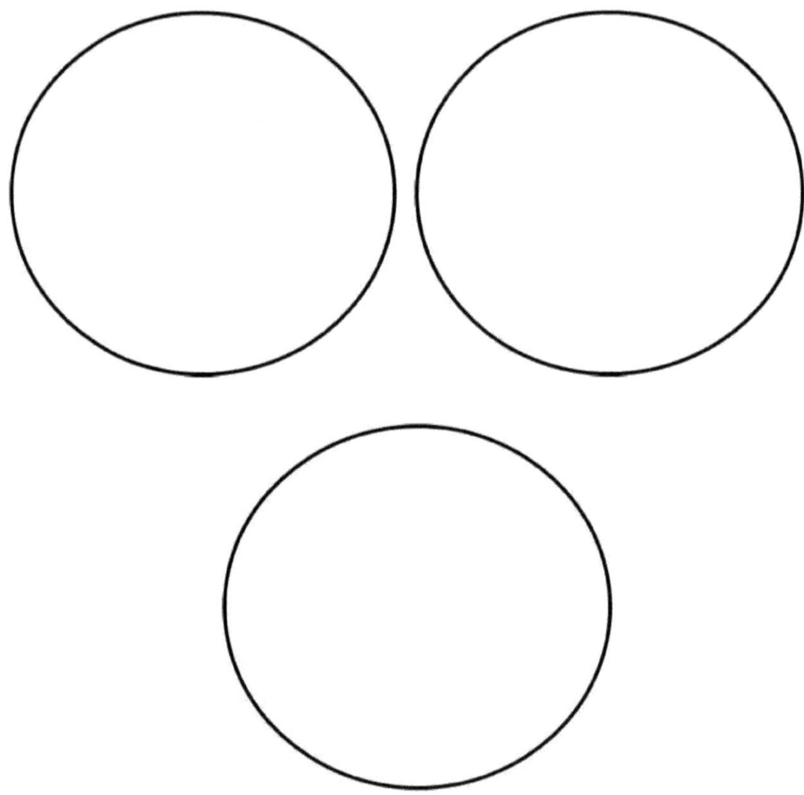

QUESTIONNAIRE

1) What are the main functions of epithelial tissue?

2) List the characteristics of epithelial lining tissue.

3) List the characteristics of glandular epithelial tissue.

4) What specialisations can the surfaces of epithelial cells acquire?

5) List the characteristics of connective tissue.

6) What is the main function of this tissue?

7) Name its main cells.

8) What are fibroblasts used for?

CHAPTER 6

ANIMAL TISSUES: MUSCULAR AND NERVOUS

Muscular tissue

Muscle tissue has elongated cells, a moderate amount of extracellular matrix and its main function is to promote body movement. The components of these cells are named differently. The cytoplasm is called sarcolemma, the cytosol is called sarcoplasm and the smooth endoplasmic reticulum is called sarcoplasmic reticulum. This tissue can be differentiated into three other types of muscle tissue: smooth, cardiac and skeletal.

Smooth muscle tissue contains long cells, thicker in the centre and tapering towards the ends (fusiform), with a single, central nucleus and no transverse striations. The cells that make up this tissue are covered by a basal lamina and are joined by a network of reticular fibres. This network allows the entire muscle to contract simultaneously. The cytoplasm of smooth muscle cells has caverns, depressions that contain Ca ions^{2+} used in the contraction process. There are also dense bodies, structures that play an important role in smooth muscle contraction, located in the cytoplasm of smooth muscle cells. These structures play an important role in the contraction process.

Cardiac muscle tissue has elongated, branched cells that are joined by intercellular junctions. Cardiac fibres have one or two centrally located nuclei and are transversely striated. They also have intercalated discs, which are highly coloured transverse lines where junctional complexes such as adhesion zonules, desmosomes and gap junctions are present. These junctions serve to unite the cells of the cardiac muscle during contraction. In addition, this muscle contains many mitochondria that are important for energy generation and secretory granules that contain the precursor molecule for atrial natriuretic peptide.

Skeletal muscle tissue is made up of bundles of long, multinucleated, cylindrical cells. In these fibres, a large number of nuclei are concentrated on the periphery. The bundles are surrounded by connective tissue called the epimysium. Subsequently, the fibre bundles

will be surrounded by the perimysium. Finally, each muscle fibre is surrounded by the endomysium. Connective tissue is responsible for holding the muscle fibres together during contraction, and it is also through it that blood vessels, lymphatic vessels and nerves penetrate the muscle.

Nervous tissue

Nervous tissue is mainly made up of little extracellular matrix, neurons and glia cells.

Neurons, also called nerve cells, conduct the nerve impulse and release neurotransmitters. These cells have the following components: dendrites, cell body or perikaryon and axon.

Glial cells represent a variety of cells that are responsible for the nutrition, protection and repair of nervous tissue. These include oligondendrocytes or Schwann cells, astrocytes, ependymal cells and microglia.

Nervous tissue can be divided into two different regions, called grey matter and white matter. Grey matter is so called because it predominantly contains neuron bodies and glia cells. The white matter, on the other hand, contains neuron extensions (axons) that are coated with a whitish material (myelin) and glial cells.The entire nervous system is lined and protected by the meninges, which are connective tissue membranes. It is also protected by the cranial box and the spinal canal.

ACTIVITIES

BLADE: TONGUE - HE

1. Under a 4X objective, make a schematic drawing of the tongue blade and identify the epithelial tissue, the connective tissue and the longitudinal and transverse muscle tissue.
2. Using a 10X objective, identify and make a schematic drawing of the muscle fibres, observing the striations of the striated skeletal muscle tissue.

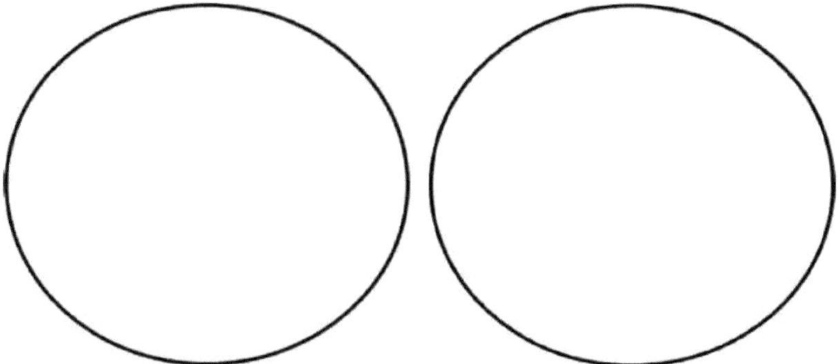

SLIDE: BONE MARROW - HE

1) Using a 10X objective, identify and draw a schematic of the neuronal bodies.

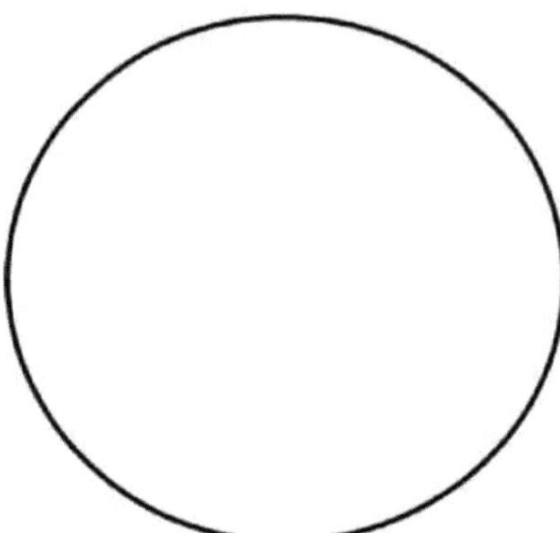

QUESTIONNAIRE

2) List the histological characteristics of smooth muscle tissue.
3) List the histological characteristics of cardiac muscle tissue.
4) List the histological characteristics of skeletal muscle tissue.
5) What is the constitution of nervous tissue?
6) What are the functions of the main cells that make up this tissue?
7) Name the cells known as glial cells.

CHAPTER 7

BONE TISSUE

Intramembranous ossification

Bone tissue is lined internally by a loose connective tissue called the endosteum. This connective tissue contains fine collagen fibres associated with active osteoblasts, resting osteoblasts, osteoclasts and osteoprogenitor cells that surround the bone trabeculae. Externally, the bone tissue is covered by a sheath of orderly dense connective tissue. Collagen fibres predominate on its outer surface, compared to the inner surface, facing the bone tissue, which is much more cellular and contains osteoprogenitor cells.

The tissue that fills the space between the bone tissue trabeculae, mesenchymal tissue, is poorly stained and has blood capillaries, sometimes with red blood cells inside, mesenchymal cells and few fibrous intercellular elements. It is whiter in sections.

The first bone tissue to appear during bone formation is called primary bone tissue. In the presence of this tissue, the bone is immature and has a bone matrix made up of bone trabeculae with numerous osteocytes arranged irregularly in the matrix, as well as many active osteoblasts and the presence of osteoclasts in the endosteum region. Compared to secondary bone tissue, primary bone tissue has a lower mineral content and a greater number of osteocytes.

The bone matrix has both organic and inorganic components. The organic part is made up of pink (acidophilic) bone trabeculae due to the predominance of thick collagen fibres, proteoglycans and glycoproteins. The inorganic part is made up of many ions, the main ones being phosphate and calcium. But bicarbonate, magnesium, potassium, sodium and citrate ions are also present.

Active osteoblasts are low cubic or prismatic cells, in the shape of a "candle flame" and well coloured. They are arranged on the surface of the tissue in a row, are seen in the endosteum, have an eccentric nucleus and basophilic cytoplasm. Their function is to synthesise the organic part of the bone matrix, osteonectin and osteocalcin. They also concentrate calcium phosphate, acting in the mineralisation of the matrix. On the other hand, inactive or resting osteoblasts are flattened cells with an elongated nucleus, located in the endosteum along with active osteoblasts.

When the bone matrix undergoes calcification, the osteoblasts become trapped in gaps inside the bone trabeculae and are called osteocytes. These cells maintain the bone matrix.

Osteoclasts are giant, multinucleated mobile cells with an irregular shape. They are found on the surface of resorbing bone trabeculae and in the innermost layer of the periosteum, close to the bone tissue. They also originate from mononucleated precursors coming from the bone marrow. Their cytoplasm is granular and may contain vacuoles, which are slightly basophilic in young osteoclasts and acidophilic in mature osteoclasts. In primary bone tissue, the osteocytes and collagen fibres are irregularly arranged, while in secondary bone tissue they are regularly distributed between the collagen fibres (lamellae).

ACTIVITIES

SLIDE: INTRAMEMBRANOUS OSSIFICATION - HE

1. Using a 10x objective, make a schematic drawing identifying periosteum, endosteum, mesenchymal tissue and bone matrix.
2. Under a 40X objective, identify and make a schematic drawing of the osteocytes, lacunae, osteoblasts and osteoclasts.
3. Using a 10X objective, identify and draw a schematic of the bone marrow with its haematopoietic tissue.

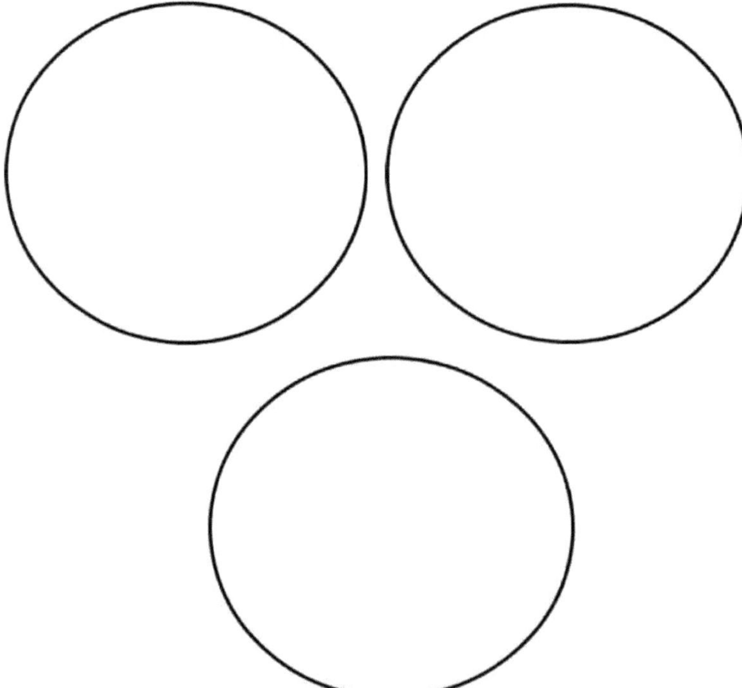

Compact Bone

Secondary or mature bone tissue is made up of collagen fibres arranged in parallel lamellae, which are concentrically arranged around channels containing vessels. This whole structure is called the Havers system or osteon.

Havers' canals are long, cylindrical canals lined by endosteum and contain vessels and nerves. It runs parallel to the major axis of the long bones.

Volkmann's canals are transverse or oblique canals that cross the bone lamellae and do not have concentric bone lamellae. They are responsible for communicating Havers' canals with each other, with the medullary cavity and with the external surface of the bone.

BLADE: WORN COMPACT BONE

1. Under a 10X objective, identify and draw a schematic diagram of Havers' system, identifying the osteocytes and Havers' canal.
2. Using the 4X objective, identify and make a schematic drawing of Volkmann's canal.

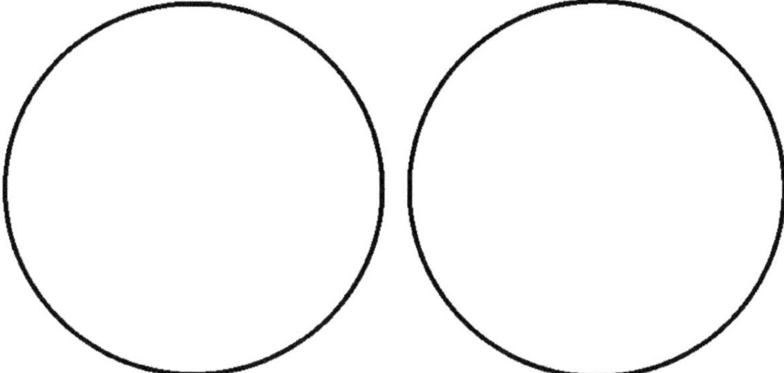

Endochondral Ossification

In membranous (or direct) ossification, the bone tissue originates directly inside the mesenchymal tissue. Undifferentiated mesenchymal cells undergo mitosis and differentiate into osteoblasts, which synthesise osteoid and become osteocytes.

Endochondral (or indirect) ossification occurs in two stages. In the first stage, the hyaline cartilage undergoes changes, the chondrocytes hypertrophy, there is a reduction in the cartilage matrix, its mineralisation and chondrocyte apoptosis. In the second stage, the sites occupied by the chondrocytes are invaded by blood capillaries and osteogenic cells. These cells differentiate into osteoblasts, which are responsible for depositing bone matrix on the calcified cartilage. In short, the mesenchymal tissue gives rise to hyaline cartilage and later the cartilage is removed and replaced by bone tissue.The regions of the epiphyseal disc are divided into the following five zones:

1. **Resting cartilage zone**: normal chondrocytes and cartilage matrix

Basophilic, i.e. unaltered hyaline cartilage.

2. **Zone of serial cartilage or proliferation**: The chondrocytes divide and form rows or columns of flattened cells.

3. **Zone of hypertrophic cartilage**: The chondrocytes in this zone are very large (hypertrophic) and continue to line up. The matrix is reduced between the hypertrophic cells.

4. Calcified cartilage zone: formed by one or two rows of empty lacunae or with degenerated chondrocytes inside due to apoptosis.

5. Zone of erosion and bone formation or ossification: Contains bone spicules with remnants of basophilic calcified cartilaginous matrix that served as a support for the beginning of bone **formation**.

deposition of acidophilic bone matrix by osteoblasts.

ACTIVITIES

FILE: KNEE - ENDOCHONDRAL OSSIFICATION - HE

1. Under a 40X objective, identify and make a schematic drawing of the endochondral ossification zones of the epiphyseal disc of a long bone.

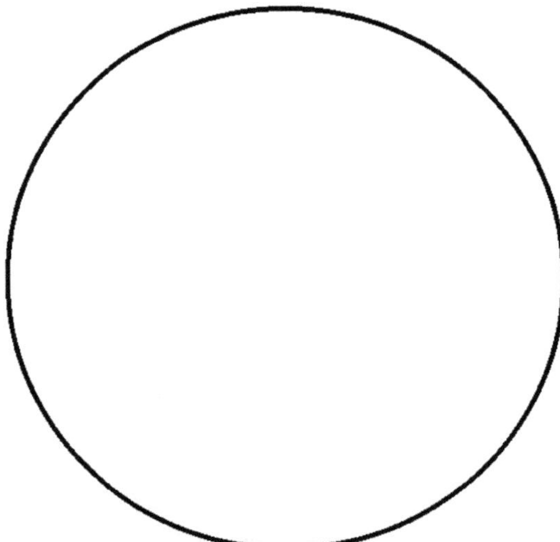

QUESTIONNAIRE

1) List the cells that make up bone tissue and their histological characteristics.
2) What are the functions of the cells mentioned in the previous exercise?
3) List the organic and inorganic constitution of the bone matrix.
4) What is the constitution and function of the periosteum and endosteum?
5) List the characteristics of primary bone tissue.
6) What is the Havers System? What is its function?
7) What is the function of the Volkmann canal?
8) What type of bone tissue contains the structures mentioned above?
9) List the five zones present in the epiphyseal disc and their respective characteristics.
10) What are the two main processes that occur in endochondral ossification?

11) What are the main functions of epithelial tissue?

12) List the characteristics of lining epithelial tissue and glandular epithelial tissue.

13) What specialisations can the surfaces of epithelial cells acquire?

14) A 7-year-old boy arrives at the hospital after falling off his bike. He complains of a lot of pain in his arm and his mother suspects it's broken. The doctor finds a bone fracture. The boy's arm is then immobilised. Describe the steps involved in repairing the bone fracture and the ossification process involved in reattaching the bone.

CHAPTER 8

CIRCULATORY SYSTEM

Large calibre arteries

The circulatory system is made up of two functional components: the blood vascular system and the lymphatic vascular system. The blood vascular system is made up of a circuit of vessels through which blood flow is maintained by the continuous pumping of the heart.

They are part of it:

A - The arterial system, which provides a distribution network from the heart to the capillaries.

B - The capillaries, which are the main sites of exchange between the tissues and the blood.

C - The venous system, which allows blood to return from the capillaries to the heart.

D - The lymphatic vascular system is a passive drainage system for returning excess extravascular fluid (lymph) back into the circulatory system.

The tissues that make up the vessel wall are represented by the following structures:

1 - Endothelium: responsible for mediating the exchanges that take place between the plasma and the interstitial fluid.

2 - Muscular tissue: represented by smooth muscle and, in a variant form, makes up the blood vessels (except capillaries and venules).

3 - Connective tissue: collagen prevents the vessel from stretching too much during its extension.

The largest calibre vessels in the circulatory system have a wall made up of:

1 - The tunica intima - made up of a layer of flattened epithelial cells (endothelium), arranged on a basal membrane; loose connective tissue (subendothelial layer) and the internal elastic limiting membrane (internal elastic limiting membrane).

2 - The *tunica media* - intermediate, of variable thickness, made up of smooth muscle fibres, elastic fibres and predominantly one of the two components mentioned above, depending on the type of vessel examined. Externally, it presents the external elastic limiting membrane.

4 -The tunica adventitia - this is the outermost of the three tunics and is made up of loose connective tissue, myelinated and amyelinated nerve fibres ("nerv/ *vasorum")* and small blood vessels (arterioles and capillaries) called "vasa *vasorum"*.

ACTIVITIES

BLADE: LARGE CALIBRE ARTERY - VERHOEFF

1. Using a 4X objective, identify and draw a schematic of the large calibre artery, identifying the tunica intima, tunica media and tunica adventitia.

2. Using the 10X objective, identify and draw a picture of the elastic fibres of the tunica media.

3. Using a 10X objective, identify and draw a picture of the *vasa vasorum* in the tunica adventitia.

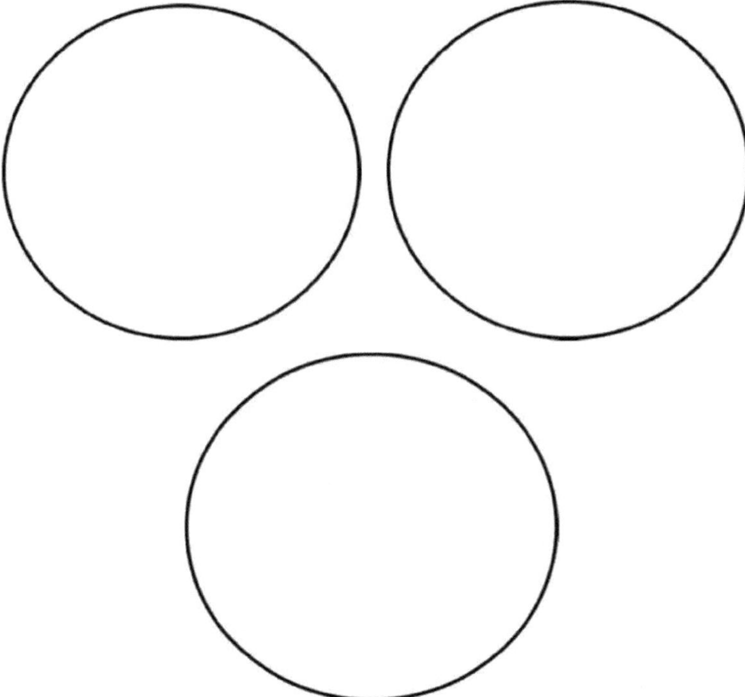

BLADE: VASCULAR NERVE BUNDLE - HE

1. Using a 10X objective, identify and make a schematic drawing of a medium calibre artery and vein. Identify the tunicae intima, media and adventitia in both the artery and vein.

2. Using a 40X objective, identify and draw a schematic diagram of a 1-, 2- and 3-cell blood capillary.

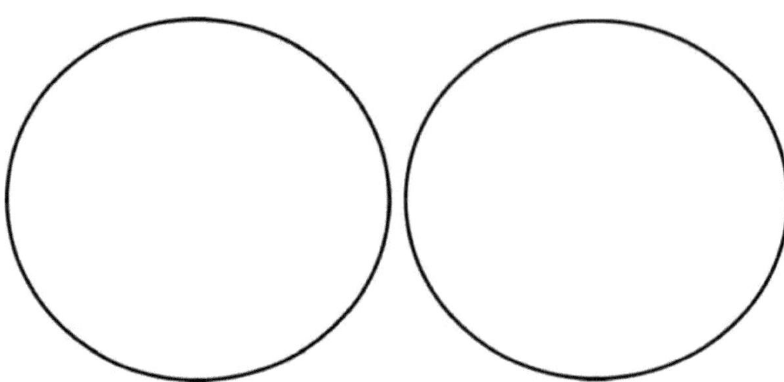

QUESTIONNAIRE

1) Explain the function of large calibre arteries or elastic arteries, correlating this with the large number of elastic laminae present in the tunica media of these arteries.

2) List the characteristics of the three tunics that make up large calibre arteries.

3) Describe the types of capillaries in terms of their structure, functional importance and occurrence.

4) Compare arterial and venous vessels of different calibres according to their constitution and thickness.

5) Relate the role of medium and large calibre arteries in the body to the composition of their tunica media

6) What is an aneurysm? Relate the disease to the tunics of the artery.

CHAPTER 9

BLOOD AND HAEMATOPOIESIS

Red blood cells

Normal red blood cells are in the shape of biconcave discs, 7 to 8p in diameter. In addition, their biconcavity increases the cell's contact surface, facilitating gas exchange. They are the most abundant cells in the blood, anucleate when adult and stain pinkish-yellow with eosin.

Platelets

Platelets, or thrombocytes, measure between 1 and 3p in diameter and are derived from the cytoplasm of megakaryocytes in the bone marrow. They have a discoid shape and no nucleus, but the cytoplasm contains mitochondria, numerous granules with different electron densities and glycogen, which is used to obtain energy for the platelet. They are coloured red and are relatively smaller than red blood cells. Platelets linked to blood clotting can be isolated or grouped together and are pinkish-red in colour. They are small because they are fragments of larger cells called megakaryocytes.

Leucocytes

Leucocytes, or white blood cells, are nucleated cells from the bone marrow that participate in the immune system. They are transported around the body via the blood and are found in the lymph, lymphoid organs and various connective tissues. Leucocytes are classified as polymorphonuclear (neutrophils, eosinophils and basophils) and monomorphonuclear (lymphocytes and monocytes). The nuclei of all leucocytes are stained purple by methylene blue.

Neutrophils

In adults under normal conditions, the neutrophil is the most abundant leucocyte, with an incidence of up to 70%, and measures 12 to 15p in diameter. The nucleus has chromatin in rod-shaped clumps or segmented into 2 to 5 lobes linked by heterochromatin filaments. The greater the number of segments, the older the cell. The cytoplasm shows a neutral reaction to haematological stains, as well as numerous small granules. The latter are made up of oxidative enzymes that promote the ingestion and destruction of microorganisms, as well as hydrolytic enzymes. Neutrophil granules are coloured salmon by a mixture of components.

Eosinophils

Eosinophils are slightly larger in diameter than neutrophils, measuring between 12 and 17p. They have a generally bilobed nuclear morphology with a chromatin bridge, with orange-red granulations in the cytoplasm stained with eosin.

Basophils

Basophils are the leucocytes with the lowest reference values in the blood - around 0% to 2%. They range in size from 10 to 15p and, under normal conditions, the nucleus has no more than two lobes and is not completely visible, being covered by coarse, dense, dark granulations in the cytoplasm, made up of acid mucopolysaccharides, histamine, heparin, serotonin and peroxidase.

Lymphocytes

Lymphocytes can be categorised as small, medium and large. Their nucleus occupies almost the entire cell and the bluish cytoplasm is more on the periphery.

Monocytes

Monocytes measure between 15 and 18p and are the largest cells in the blood. The nucleus is quite irregular and can be seen in a **lobulated, rhiniform or U-shaped** form. **The cytoplasm of** normal **monocytes** is blue-grey in colour, with small and few azurophilic granules containing the enzyme esterase.

SLIDE: BLOOD SMEAR

ACTIVITIES:

Before you start looking through the microscope, make sure the smear is facing upwards, then place it on the microscope slide, as this slide is not protected by a coverslip.

1. Under a 100X objective, identify and make a schematic drawing of the cells: red blood cells, lymphocytes, neutrophils, eosinophils, basophils, monocytes and platelets.

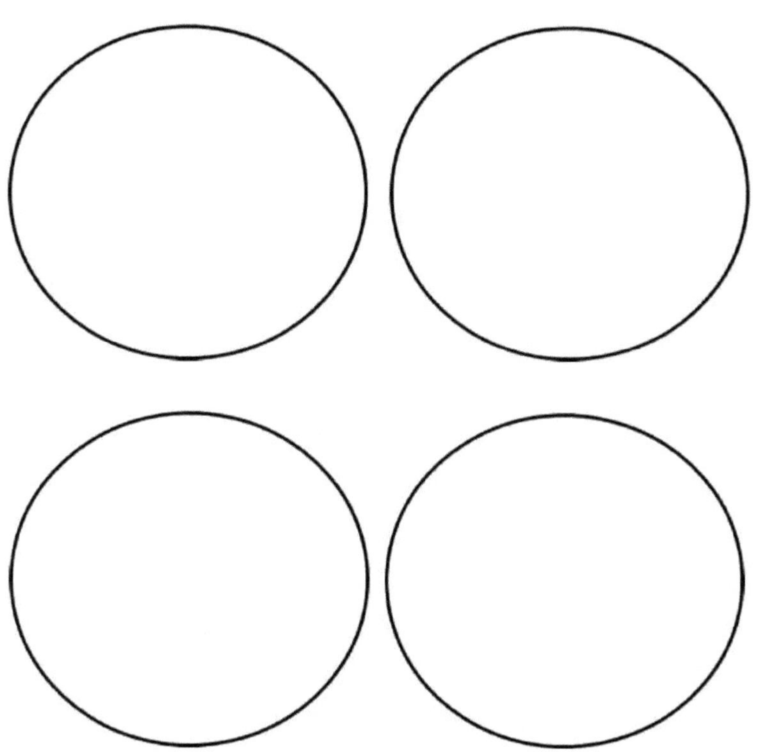

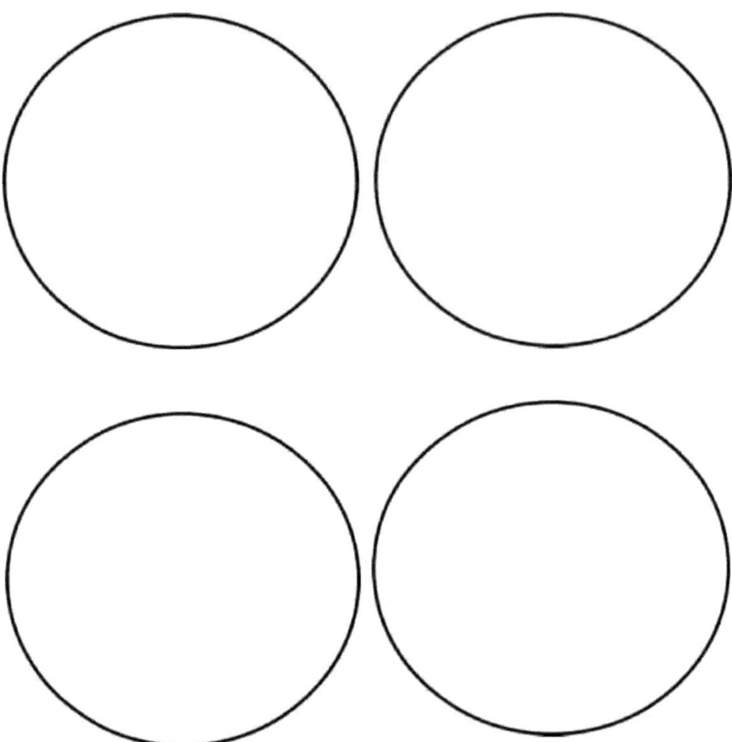

QUESTIONNAIRE:

1) Differentiate between red blood cells and leucocytes.
2) What is haematopoietic tissue? Where is it located?
3) What is the difference between myeloid and lymphoid lineages?
4) What are the granules in the cytoplasm of a basophile made up of?
5) Name one function of each cell: RBCs, Platelets, Neutrophils, Eosinophils, Basophils, Lymphocytes, Monocytes.
6) What are the progenitor cells of red blood cells, platelets, neutrophils and lymphocytes?
7) For each type of blood cell, list a disease when the cell is increased in number and when it is reduced in number.
8) What is the relationship between blood cells and the lymphatic system?

CHAPTER 10

LYMPHATIC SYSTEM: THYMUS AND LYMPH NODES

Timo

The thymus has a dense connective tissue capsule with fatty tissue and blood vessels. This organ consists of two lobes, which are divided into lobules by septa formed through the capsule. There are no afferent or efferent lymphatic vessels in the thymus. Each lobe has a cortex (darker region) and a medulla (lighter region) and are interconnected by the medulla. The population of cells (thymocytes) in the cortex is greater than in the medulla, which explains its darker colour. The cells that go to the medulla come from the cortex, and the lymphocytes that reach the cortex originate in the bone marrow or foetal liver. In the cortex, the cells acquire immunological competence and then head for the medulla, which in turn throws them into the lumen of the post-capillary venules.

T lymphocytes are always travelling through these regions in a movement called lymphocyte recirculation. In the thymus, there are epithelial reticular cells, macrophages and dendritic cells (antigen presenting cells). There are three types of epithelial reticular cells in the cortex and three types in the medulla. There is only one type of epithelial reticular cell, type VI, located in the thymic or Hassall's corpuscles, which characterise the thymus and are present in the medulla. These corpuscles are made up of a group of epithelial reticular cells organised in concentric layers and joined by numerous desmosomes. The epithelial reticular cells that form the thymic corpuscles are thought to be in the process of degeneration, and calcification of the corpuscle may occur. The thymus has two origins: its epithelial reticular cells originate from the endoderm and the lymphocytes originate from the haematopoietic tissue (mesoderm) of the bone marrow.

Lymph node

The lymph node is surrounded by a capsule of dense, unmoulded connective tissue, continuous with the surrounding tissue, including unilocular adipose tissue. The capsule is thicker at the hilum and emits trabeculae into the organ, carrying blood vessels. The supporting framework of the lymph node is made up of trabeculae rich in collagen fibres and the network of reticular fibres of the lymphoid tissue.

The lymph node parenchyma is divided into the cortex, which is peripheral, and the medulla, which is central and close to the hilum. The cortex can be subdivided into the superficial cortex, which is more external, and the deep cortex (or paracortex), which underlies the anterior cortex.

- Cortical region: this is made up of loose lymphoid tissue, which forms the subcapsular and peritrabecular sinuses, and lymphatic nodules or follicles which may have germinal centres. B lymphocytes are the predominant cells.

- Paracortical region: there are no lymph nodes and T lymphocytes predominate, along with reticular cells and some plasma cells and macrophages.

- Medullary region: consists of the medullary cords, formed mainly by B lymphocytes, and the medullary sinuses, which separate the cords. Plasma cells are generally more numerous in the medullary region than in the cortical region.

ACTIVITIES

BLADE: THYMUS - HE

1. Using a 4X objective, identify and draw a schematic of the capsule and lobes. From one lobe, identify and draw a schematic of the cortical region and the medullary region.
2. Under a 40X objective, identify and make a schematic drawing of: Hassall's corpuscle, lymphocytes and reticular cells.

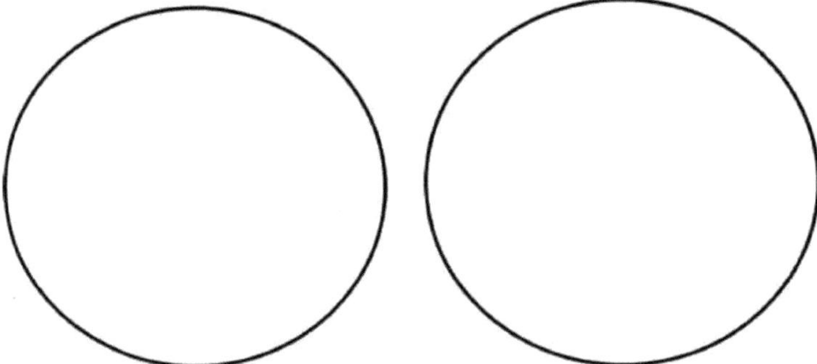

SLIDE: LYMPH NODE - HE

1. Using a 4x lens, identify and draw a schematic diagram of the capsule, cortical, paracortical and medullary regions.
2. Under the 10x objective, in the cortical region, identify and draw a schematic drawing of the regions: lymph node, subcapsular sinus and peritrabecular sinus.
3. Under a 10x objective, in the medullary region, identify and make a schematic drawing of the regions: medullary cords and medullary sinuses.

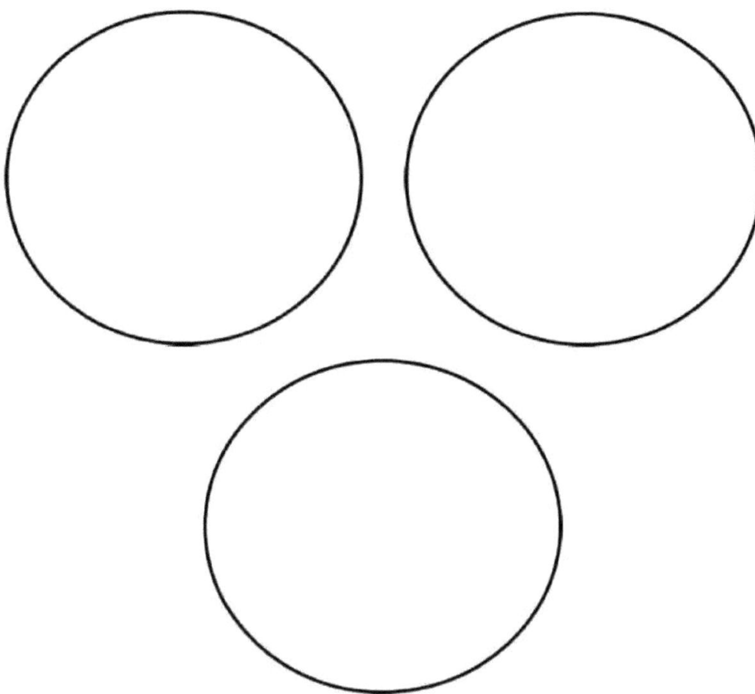

QUESTIONNAIRE

1) Histologically differentiate the cortical and medullary regions of the thymus.
2) What is Hassal's corpuscle? What is its function?
3) What are the embryonic origins of the thymus and which cells represent them?
4) Differentiate the regions (cortical, paracortical and medullary) of the lymph node.

CHAPTER 11

LYMPHATIC SYSTEM: SPLEEN AND MALT

Spleen

The spleen, the largest lymphoid organ in the body, plays an essential role in the body's defence and also acts as the body's main destroyer of red blood cells. This organ is rich in cells with a phagocytic function, contributing to a rapid immunological response to antigens that enter the bloodstream.

It has a thick capsule of dense, unmoulded connective tissue. This capsule is lined by a simple pavement epithelial tissue, also called mesothelium. Connective tissue septa derived from the capsule penetrate the spleen parenchyma (splenic pulp), carrying blood vessels into the organ. Histologically, the splenic pulp is subdivided into white pulp and red pulp:

- The white pulp corresponds to the lymph nodes, which are organised in a cylindrical sheath with several layers of lymphocytes surrounded by a central artery. B lymphocytes predominate in this region.
- The red pulp consists of a loose lymphoid tissue made up of splenic cords (Billroth's cords) that are separated by sinusoids. As well as containing lymphocytes (B and T), it also has a vast number of other cells, such as red blood cells, macrophages, granulocytes and so on.

The region of lymphocytes at the junction of the periarterial lymphoid sheath and the red pulp is known as the marginal zone. This zone has an important immune function, as it surrounds numerous antigens from the bloodstream.

Another region of the spleen is the hilum, which is responsible for allowing nerves and vessels to reach the organ.

MALT

The extensive lymphatic tissue of the mucous membranes is called MALT (mucosa-associated lymphoid tissue). MALT is made up of lymphoid tissue (mainly T lymphocytes) and is present in the mucous membranes of various systems of the body, such as the mucous membranes of the digestive, respiratory and urinary systems. It is made up of clusters of lymphoid tissue situated in strategic locations, which are generally subject to the entry of antigens (molecules or microorganisms) from the outside. In some regions of the body, this cluster of lymphatic tissue generates organs such as Peyer's patches located in the ileum and tonsils.

ACTIVITIES

LAMINA: SMALL INTESTINE - ILEUM (MALT)

1. Under a 4X objective, identify and draw a schematic diagram of the regions of mucosa-associated lymphoid tissue - MALT (Peyer's patch).

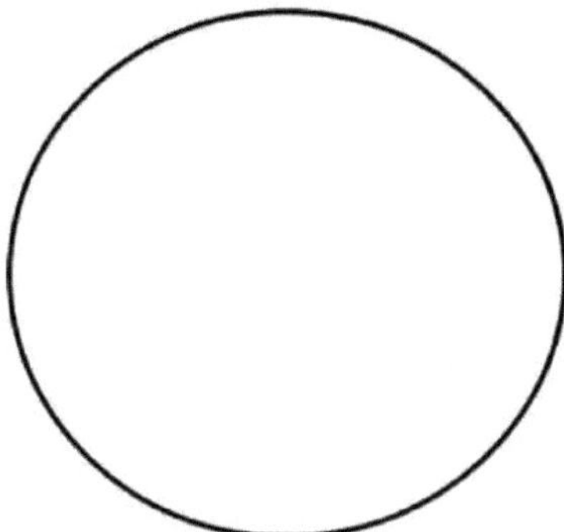

BLADE: SPLEEN -HE

1. Using a 4X objective, identify and draw a schematic diagram of the capsule, septum, white pulp and red pulp.
2. Under a 10X objective, identify and make a schematic drawing of the white pulp showing the lymph node and the central artery.
3. Under a 40X objective, identify and make a schematic drawing of the sinusoids and splenic cords.

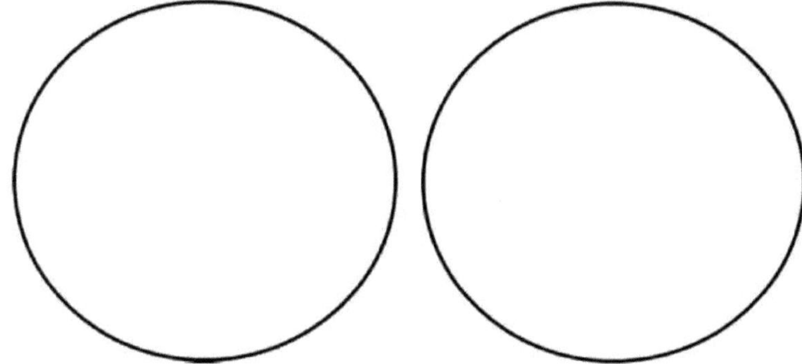

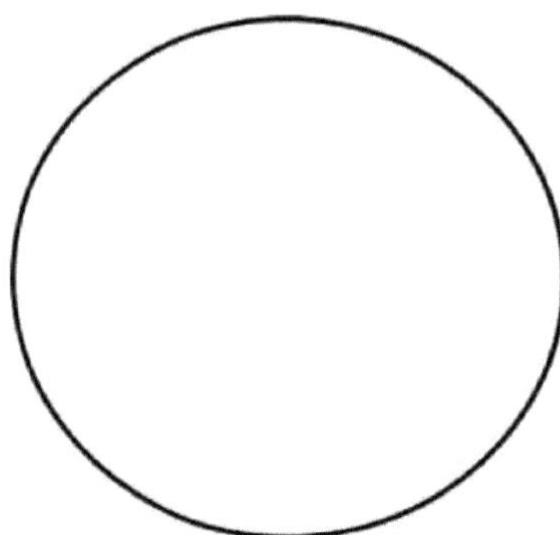

QUESTIONNAIRE

1) Describe the spleen histologically.

2) Explain the lymphatic circulation within the spleen.

3) Where is the marginal zone found? Describe its importance in the immune system.

4) Name the composition of MALT.

5) Apart from the intestine and tonsils, what other organs do we find MALT in?

6) Mr Sofrônico has had pulmonary tuberculosis for 40 years. At his last consultation, he was also diagnosed with ganglion tuberculosis. This disease affects the lymph nodes, also known as lymph nodes. On the histology of this lymph node, select the correct option:

a) It has parenchyma divided into white pulp and red pulp b) In the medullary region it has splenic cords and splenic sinuses.
7) It is classified as a primary lymphoid organ
8) Its parenchyma is divided into cortical, paracortical and medullary regions. e) It has reticular epithelial cells and Hassal's corpuscle.

7) Lancelot, 55, a long-time drinker, with hepatosplenic schistosomiasis. Schistosomiasis is a parasitic disease transmitted by planorbids (snails). As it is a parasitic disease, Mr Lancelot's blood count is expected to show an increase in which blood cell?

a) Plate
b) Neutrophil
c) Eosinophilic
d) Haematia
e) Megakaryotic

CHAPTER 12

RESPIRATORY SYSTEM

Trachea

The trachea is lined internally by a pseudostratified cylindrical ciliated epithelium with goblet cells, resting on a lamina propria of loose connective tissue, which is richly vascularised, humidifying and warming the air. Between the mucosa and submucosa is a concentration of elastic fibres that can only be seen with special techniques. Just below it are seromucous glands whose ducts open into the tracheal lumen.

It has C-shaped cartilage pieces that are lined with perichondrium and joined posteriorly by fibroelastic ligaments and smooth muscle bundles. The cartilaginous rings prevent the wall from collapsing. The trachea is lined externally by a loose connective tissue, constituting the adventitial layer, which connects the organ to adjacent tissues.

Lungs

Most of the lamina of the lung mass is made up of alveoli, which are normally filled with air. The bronchi are tubes that carry air into the lungs and are lined by a respiratory epithelium, beneath which is a lamina propria surrounded by a layer of smooth muscle fibres, and more peripherally by plates of hyaline cartilage. They branch off and form tubes called bronchioles.

The bronchioles branch out until they reach structures where their epithelium is paved, and are then called alveolar ducts. The alveolar ducts begin the actual respiratory portion. They are long, tortuous ducts that end in alveoli or alveolar sacs (groups of alveoli that open into a common chamber).

Bronchi

- Mucosa: ciliated to simple cylindrical pseudostratified epithelium with goblet cells. Lamina propria of loose connective tissue rich in elastic fibres.

- Layer of smooth muscle tissue: spirally arranged muscle bundles that completely encircle the bronchus.
- Connective tissue layer: containing seromucous glands that open their ducts into the bronchial lumen.
- Hyaline cartilage plates: these appear as islands between connective tissue rich in elastic fibres. This connective layer, often called the adventitial layer, continues with the connective fibres of the adjacent lung tissue.

Bronchioles

The mucosa begins with a simple cylindrical ciliated epithelium with a few goblet cells and changes to a simple cubic intermittently ciliated epithelium supported by a thin lamina propria of loose connective tissue rich in elastic fibres. Layer of smooth muscle tissue very well developed and arranged helicordally.

Terminal bronchioles

They are the last portions of the bronchial tree. They are similar in structure to the bronchioles, but have a thinner wall, lined internally by a low columnar or cubic epithelium with ciliated and non-ciliated cells. They also have Clara cells, which are non-ciliated and have secretory granules in their apical portions.

Respiratory bronchioles

They form the transition between the conductive and respiratory portions. They are lined by cubic epithelium over fibroelastic connective tissue and smooth muscle. This segment is characterised by alveoli in its walls. It also contains Clara cells in its epithelium.

Alveoli

Sacs lined by simple flat epithelium supported by connective tissue rich in elastic fibres, richly supplied by capillaries. The common alveolar wall between two alveoli is the interalveolar septum. The interalveolar septum is made up of:

- Type I pneumocyte: also called alveolar pavement cell, it has a flattened nucleus and is separated from each other; the cytoplasm is very thin and has desmosomes connecting adjacent cells. Its main function is to form a barrier of minimal thickness to allow gas exchange and at the same time prevent the passage of liquid.
- Type II pneumocyte: also called septal cells, these are rounded cells that always remain under the basal membrane of the alveolar epithelium, as part of that epithelium. The nucleus is larger and more vesicular and the cytoplasm is not thinned and appears vacuolised under light microscopy. They produce surfactant which reduces the surface tension of the alveoli.
- Capillary endothelial cells: these are the most numerous and have the most elongated nucleus. The endothelium is continuous, not frenestrated.

Honeycomb bag

Group of alveoli that open into a common space.

Pleura

Serosa lining the lungs: mesothelium and loose connective tissue rich in elastic fibres. Only the visceral leaflet is seen on the slide.

ACTIVITIES

BLADE: TRACHEA - HE

1. Using a 4X objective, make a schematic drawing of the respiratory epithelium, connective tissue, seromucous glands, perichondrium, hyaline cartilage and adventitia.
2. Under a 40X objective, make a schematic drawing of the hyaline cartilage, highlighting the chondrocytes in the lacunae and the cartilaginous matrix.
3. Under a 40X objective, make a schematic drawing of the respiratory epithelial tissue indicating the presence of ciliated column cells and goblet cells.

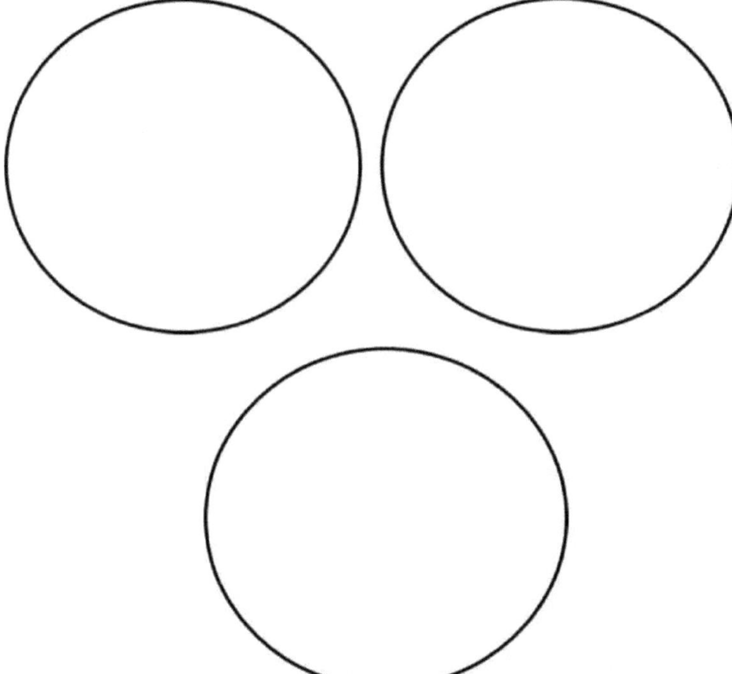

SLIDE: LUNG-HE

1. Using a 4X objective, identify and draw a schematic of the bronchus.
2. Under a 10X objective, identify and draw a schematic drawing of: terminal bronchioles and respiratory bronchioles, alveolar duct and alveoli.
3. Using a 10X objective, identify and draw a schematic of the alveolar duct, alveolar sac and alveoli.

4. Under a 40X objective, identify and make a schematic drawing of the interalveolar septum with its constituent cells (type I pneumocyte, type II pneumocyte and capillary endothelial cells).

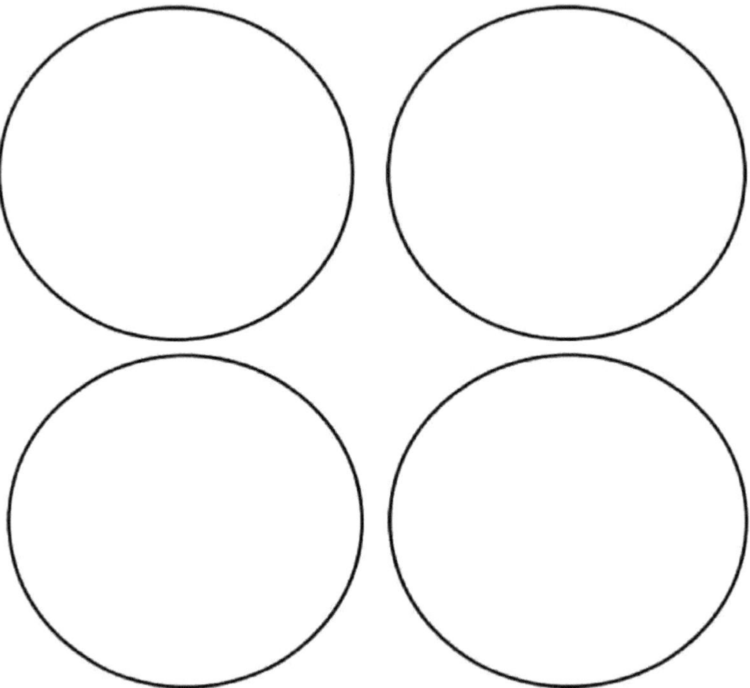

QUESTIONNAIRE

1) Why do the larynx, trachea and bronchi have cartilaginous parts?

2) What type of epithelium is found in the mucosa of the trachea? Describe the cell found in this epithelium.

3) What are intralveolar septa? What are they for?

4) Name the importance of Clara's cells.

5) What is the substance that facilitates the expansion of the alveoli during inspiration and prevents them from collapsing during expiration? Which cell secretes it?

6) Explain what the interalveolar wall is and which cells make it up.

7) Name a function of pneumocyte I and pneumocyte II.

8) Research the histological constitution of the Pleura and its functions.

9) In a patient who smokes, what histological changes occur in the respiratory system?

CHAPTER 13

URINARY SYSTEM

Kidney

Encapsulated organ divided into cortex and medulla. Hilum with vessels (renal artery and renal vein) and nerves. It contains calyces that come together to form the renal pelvis, the upper, dilated part of the ureter. The functional unit of the kidney is the nephron:

Renal or Malpighian corpuscle

It is formed by a tangle of capillaries (Malpighi's glomerulus) surrounded by Bowman's capsule, which has two leaflets: visceral, next to the capillaries, formed by podocytes; and parietal, of simple pavement epithelium. There is a space between them, the capsular or Bowman's space. Each corpuscle has 2 poles: vascular, through which the efferent arteriole enters and the vessels that drain the glomerulus exit; and urinary, where the proximal convoluted tubule arises. In addition to endothelial cells and podocytes, glomeruli contain mesangial cells, found in the spaces between the capillaries.

Renal tubules

- Proximal convoluted tubule: the cells have strongly acidophilic basal cytoplasm due to numerous elongated mitochondria. The apical cytoplasm has microvilli, which form a brush border and few nuclei. They are found in the cortex.
- Henle's loop: divided into descending and ascending parts, with a thick part similar to the distal convoluted tubule and a thin part made up of simple pavement epithelium. Predominantly medullary.
- Distal convoluted tubule: its cells are smaller (greater number of nuclei in each cross-section) than those of the proximal convoluted tubule, do not have a brush border and are less acidophilic. It is lined by a simple cubic epithelium and is also found in the cortical region. The part that passes adjacent to the vascular pole of the Malpighian corpuscle forms the macula densa.

- Collecting tubules: the thinnest collecting tubules are lined with cubic epithelium and, as they merge and approach the papillae, their cells become taller, until they become cylindrical. At the same time, the diameter of the tube increases. Throughout their length, the collecting ducts are made up of cells with cytoplasm that is weakly stained with eosin and whose intercellular boundaries are clear. These cells are clear under the electron microscope and very poor in organelles. They are found in both the medullary and cortical regions.

Bladder

The bladder and urinary tract store the urine formed by the kidneys for some time and conduct it outwards. The calyx, pelvis, ureter and bladder have the same basic structure, although the wall gradually thickens towards the bladder.

In the mucosa we can see the transitional epithelium and the lamina propria of connective tissue which varies from loose to dense. The apical membrane of an emptied bladder has globose cells, and when full, flattened cells. The tunica muscularis is made up of three not very well defined layers of smooth muscle: internal and external longitudinal and middle circular. The adventitia has fibrous connective tissue and the upper part of the bladder is covered by a serous membrane (peritoneum). The urinary bladder may or may not have folds depending on the volume of urine stored.

ACTIVITIES

BLADE: KIDNEY - HE

1. Using the lowest magnification lens, identify and draw a schematic of the medullary and cortical regions of the kidney.
2. Under a 40X objective, identify the following in the cortical region: glomerulus, macula densa, Bowman's capsule, distal and proximal convoluted tubule.
3. Under a 40X objective, identify the mesangial cells and podocytes in the glomerulus. Also identify the visceral and parietal regions of the glomerular capsule.

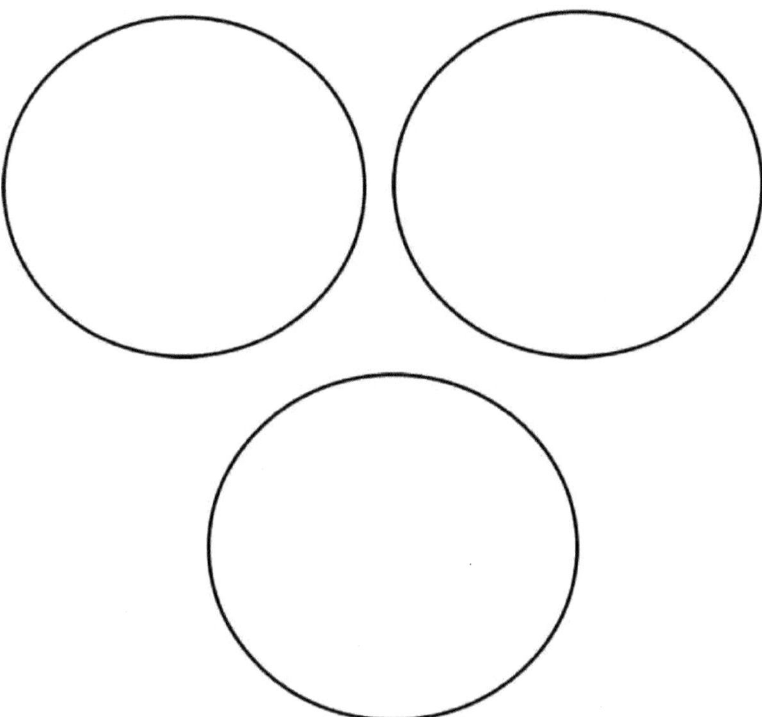

BLADE: BLADDER-HE

1. Under a 4X objective, identify and make a schematic drawing of the epithelium, lamina propria, muscular layers and serous layer.

2. At higher magnification, make a schematic drawing of the transitional epithelium of the bladder.

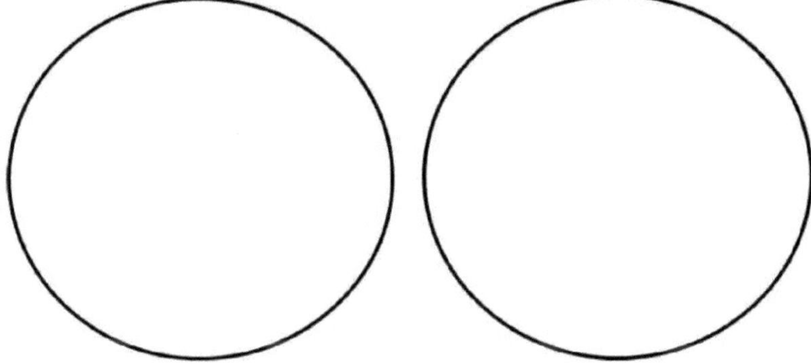

QUESTIONNAIRE

1) Describe the formation of urine, relating it to the morphology of the structures responsible.

2) Where are the mesangial cells found and what are their functions? 3) What are the constituents of the juxtaglomerular apparatus and what is its importance?

4) What is the epithelium of the ureter, bladder and urethra?

5) Mrs Xantipa, 50, has a history of systemic arterial hypertension. It is known that this disease can compromise the functioning of different organs. Concerned about this situation, the doctor ordered some tests. The result of one of these tests contained the following description: *"Presence of capsule with dense connective tissue. Organ divided into cortex and medulla. Malpighian pyramids, papillae and medullary rays preserved. Large number of Malpighi corpuscles in the* ***cortical region. Organ without considerable damage."***

Which organisation is this result about?

A) Timo

B) Adrenal

C) Lymph node

D) Kidney

E) Spleen

6) After some tests, Mr Policarpo Quaresma was told that his kidneys were starting to lose their function due to obesity and diabetes. On the subject of the kidney, tick the TRUE box.

A) The mesangial cells present in the glomerulus are an important component of the glomerular filtration barrier, preventing the passage of proteins into the blood.

B) The medullary region of the kidney contains the Malpighian corpuscle, proximal and distal convoluted tubule and medullary rays and vessels.

C) Bowman's capsule is formed by a visceral leaflet made up of pavement cells and a parietal leaflet made up of podocytes.

D) Podocytes produce renin, which is involved in regulating blood pressure.

E) Each renal corpuscle has a vascular pole through which the afferent arteriole enters and the efferent arteriole leaves, and a urinary pole where the proximal convoluted tubule begins.

BIBLIOGRAPHICAL REFERENCES

CORMACK, D. H. **Fundamentos de Histologia**. 2. ed. Rio de Janeiro: Guanabara Koogan, 2003.

JUNQUEIRA, L.C.; CARNEIRO J. **Basic Histology** - 12ª Ed. 2013.
Guanabara Koogan, 2013.

MOORE, KEITH L.; PERSAUD, T. V. N.; TORCHIA, MARK G. **Basic Embryology** - 8th Ed. Elsevier. 2013 .

TOLOSA, E. M. C.; RODRIGUES, C. J.; BEHMER, O. A. **Manual of techniques for normal and**

pathological histology. 2. ed. Barueri: Manole, 2003.

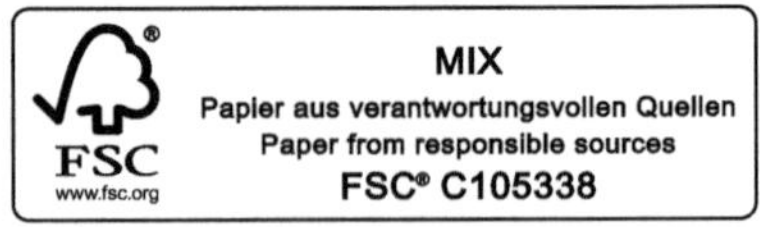

Printed by Books on Demand GmbH, Norderstedt / Germany